THE BODY RECOMPOSITION MANUAL

A GUIDE TO LOSE FAT, BUILD MUSCLE, AND LIVE A HEALTHIER LIFE:

An Effective Way To Get Fit

Disclaimer:

This book is not intended as a substitute for the medical advice of physicians. The reader should regularly consult a physician in matters relating to his/her health and particularly with respect to any symptoms that may require diagnosis or medical attention. The authors and publisher advise readers to take full responsibility for their safety and know their limits. Before practicing the skills described in this book, be sure that your equipment is well maintained, and do not take risks beyond your level of experience, aptitude, training, and comfort level.

Copyright © 2020 by ClubForFitness

ISBN: 9798684351297

Written by Charan G

All rights reserved. This book or parts thereof may not be reproduced in any form, stored in any retrieval system, or transmitted in any form by any means .

For permission requests, write to the publisher, at
"Attention: Permission Coordinator,"
at the email address below:
contactus@clubforfitness.com

TABLE OF CONTENTS

Book Description..1

Introduction...3

Chapter 1: Getting Started with Body Recomposition...........................5

Chapter 2: Nutrition for Body Recomposition.....................................11

Chapter 3: Training for Body Recomposition......................................35

Chapter 4: Sleep For Body Recomposition..49

Chapter 5: Supplements For Body Recomposition..............................55

Chapter 6: Maintaining your Body Muscle so you don't lose it, even over 50..65

Chapter 7: Mistakes of Body Recomposition and how to avoid them...71

Conclusion...75

Do You Want To Sign up In Our 12-Week Program?.........................77

But, Who Am I?...79

References...81

BOOK DESCRIPTION

Do you want to be fit?
Do you want to gain muscle?

Do you want to be healthy?

If you answered YES to the questions, then this is the right book for you. Many people start off great with their exercises and eating plan but then quickly fall off of it. This is a common problem because we live in a society that expects instant results. It takes time to lose weight and get in shape, although you can begin this process in as little as seven days. You have to be ready to commit to weight loss and do what it takes to reduce weight. The weight isn't going to come off on its own; you have to do some work. If you go into it thinking that there's some magic bullet, you're going to be disappointed in your results.

Excessive weight can definitely be an obstacle in life. This is simply the harsh reality. Although you don't want to give people the time of day who treat you any different, it's a weird world out there and sometimes it's just easier to not have an extra thing that people can judge you on, sigh.

You also have to be ready for at least some moderate activity. You need to move to keep your metabolism high which makes it easier to burn calories and keep the weight from coming back. If you're not going to be active, it will be tougher to see any sustained weight loss because your body simply needs movement for you to be successful.

You also can't lose weight on your own and you have to look to a support system to help you out. A good support system is essential – the stronger it is, the easier it will be to accomplish your goals. Your family and your friends, and anyone who is undertaking the same journey as you, will certainly play an essential role in your success.

This book will show you:

- Getting Started with Body Recomposition
- Who is Eligible for Body Recomposition?
- When Does an Exercise Stimulate a Muscle?
- General Motivation Ideas Success Tips
- Body Recomposition Mindset
- Nutrition for Body Recomposition
- The Best Diet for Body Recomposition
- Training for Body Recomposition
- Strength Training Program
- Maintaining your Body Muscle so you don't lose it, even over 50
- Mistakes of Body Recomposition and How to Avoid Them

There's just too much that goes on with you emotionally when you try to lose weight. If you don't have anyone there to back you up, your chances of failure are that much greater. A good support system can make a world of difference. With a great support system, you'll have the incentive you need to lose weight and you'll get that motivation which will help you stick with it.

Having goals will give you something to strive for. It might be to lose 15 pounds in a couple of months or be able to run several miles or even a marathon. Whatever you want to do, you need to write it down and make goals a part of your routine as they help keep you on track.

Get Your Copy Now!

INTRODUCTION

Body Recomposition is basically the process to lose fat and gain muscle at the same time instead of bulking first then cutting later or cutting first or bulking later. This process is extremely helpful for beginners who want to lose fat but also to gain muscle because neither do they have enough muscle to support a cut nor low enough fat to support a bulk. This process is also extremely beneficial for people stuck in the "skinny fat" body composition.

Skinny fat is the condition where you have little muscle and a more than little fat mass and what ends up happening is you look skinny with a shirt on but when you remove clothes, the little muscle that you have is not able to shape your fat properly and you end up looking sloppy, weak and fat. So if you are skinny fat, instead of getting more fatter and then cutting or getting even skinnier and then bulking, you can just skip these steps with body recomposition and gain muscle and lose fat at the same time which will result in you looking better slowly over time but will not give you any health risks. For example, if you start bulking at skinny fat you will gain much fat and become obese which will cause heart diseases, high cholesterol and many other problems. This book will explain everything you need to know about body recomposition. Without further ado let's get started.

CHAPTER 1:

Getting Started with Body Recomposition

Body weight workouts may be perfect for weight reduction and maintaining the strength you already have, however if you're serious about body recomposition, you'll need a gym with a squat rack, a bench, a barbell, and a place for pull-ups, chin-ups, and dips to be the most effective.

Since we're trying to build realistic strength and height, we're going to do a ton of full-body workout workouts that target several muscle groups at once.

They're more effective, they generate solid growth and relaxation, and they're going to keep you healthy. What is it?

Yeah, when you waste all the time performing dumb isolation workouts on weight machines (ugh), you're just working certain particular muscles and not working any of the stabilizer muscles (because the computer is doing all the stabilization work). On the other side, as you perform joint workouts like barbell squats, you practice pretty much every muscle in the body, setting yourself up to stay healthy and safe from injury.

Who is eligible for body recomposition?

First, we have to understand that building muscle and losing fat are two different processes and they can absolutely happen at the same time. If someone is saying it otherwise then they are lying or are misinformed. Just the degree or rate at which you will be able to achieve body recomposition gets harder or slower.

Newbies

This is an obvious one. People who are new to exercise and following a good eating plan are surely going to get results even if they put half-ass efforts. This is because as a new lifter your body has never experience this type of resistance before. We will further discuss how to exactly do it later.

Trainees returning after a break or injury

When you take a break from the gym or you are forced to take a break from the gym due to an injury, and you return to the gym later you have the same tendencies to build muscle and lose fat like a newbie. We have to understand that when you don't train your muscles your body thinks you are not using them anymore and therefore use the energy not to conserve the muscles and use it somewhere else and therefore you lose strength and size. But when you return to the gym again your muscles remember the patterns or movements of the exercises again and build the muscle back fairly quickly.

Overweight individuals

If you are already overweight you can literally go all out on your workouts because your fat is already available to give you the necessary energy to build muscle and you can start eating at a deficit to lose the fat which we'll discuss later.

People on performance enhancing drugs

Body Recomposition already works just fine but with PEDs and especially anabolic steroids your ability to gain muscle and lose fat increases greatly.

When does an exercise stimulate a muscle?

Stimulating reps will only be counted in full unless the movement generates maximum motor unit activation for the functioning muscle community, which typically implies that the muscle group needs to be the restricting factor for the movement. But certain workouts require different muscle types, and not all of them work equally well. For example, squats are likely to stimulate the quadriceps to the full since they are a restricting force but are likely to leave some stimulating reps in the tank for functioning hip extenders (adductor magnus and gluteus maximus), particularly when typical high bar squat variants are used.

At the end, how the activity activates the muscle must be decided by an appreciation of the biomechanics of the movement and not by whether it has historically been used in the routines for that portion of the body. The use of multi-joint activities can still contribute to some uncertainty, but that is an issue that we will need to deal with if we are to profit from utilizing them.

How to Stay Motivated to Achieve Desired Muscle Mass?

Have some days where you feel like you're not moving anywhere? The mere idea of getting to head to the gym lets you think about hundreds about options to persuade yourself not to participate. Egg White and Protein Powder Shake, helps you shape something a bit naughtier. You may not be isolated.

General Motivation Ideas Success Tips

- You need to report results and ensure if your contributions are compensated. It can support you in the long run and figure out what works for you and what doesn't work for you. Document your weight on a weekly or regular basis for a weekly average.

- Don't get distracted by the day you're x pounds and then day two you're x pounds + 4. Body weight is fluctuating with diet and drink. Report the routine and the full raises.

- Not only do you want to break your old numbers, it will help you spot some plateaus early on.

- Posters & Development Pictures There are two styles of posters that you might use to hold your mind centered. A snapshot of the first time you began on the side of the current shot. You may even share a image of somebody you aspire to look like. Second, you should purchase inspiration posters that have words or poems to inform you about what you're striving for.

- Note that we're people, so if you have a dishonest lunch, just apply that to the normal consumption. When I get a dishonest lunch, I make sure I make a pass to the gym, clears the mind

- Listening to the music that you want and loving listening to can help keep you focused. Remember to mix things with each other once in a while. Listening to the same music all the time would wind up tedious will potentially have a reverse impact.

- Find Workouts & Body Sections You Enjoy Have a Special Day? Or a fun workout, huh? This also can benefit when it comes to the timing of the exercise.

Body Recomposition Mindset

Why do people avoid doing something they know would be good for them?

These ideas, and variations on them, conspire to limit the chances of someone's success before they even start work.

This is called a fixed mindset. It means that people believe they can determine in advance how successful they will be at any endeavor.

The common theme in all these ideas is that the person thinks they can tell in advance how successful they will be at something before they try to do it!

People with fixed mindsets accept huge limitations on their potential before they even try to do something.

It means that one will only find out how successful they can be by working persistently at something.

People who have a growth mindset take on a new task believing "It will be difficult, but I can do this" When you have a growth mindset you approach the task knowing it may be difficult, but you are committed to giving it your best shot.

If you have lost control or simply fancied something that you couldn't resist just accept it and move on, remember you're in control. Many people eat more because they are unhappy, so whilst they aren't getting any closer to their goals and are still overweight it can cause them to be upset further and to keep eating which is a never-ending cycle of emotions that gets you nowhere.

As you know, you will not lose weight overnight so it's good to keep a mind-set that every day counts even if you can't see it on the scales. Just think of it as one big step closer even if it feels like a small step. I would advise you to not weigh yourself every day as this may put you off and any progress may seem like it's happening too slow. Stick to once a week at the same time in the morning. If you do weight yourself at different times, do not be alarmed if you seem to of put on weight as it can and will fluctuate during the day and throughout the week. This is because of things you consume and how your body handles them.

People may make fun of you for choosing to exercise and diet, they may not believe in you for whatever reason. This may be because they could not imagine themselves changing their lifestyle in such a way so in their eyes you must also fail at it. Shrug it off and continue as normal, and you will be the one laughing when you reach your goals. It's not an issue what other people think as it's your own actions that dictates your outcome. To achieve this, you need to let go of all your fears that could make it harder for you and just concentrate on the end result.

Sometimes when you are doing well you may treat yourself a little too much and then it backfires, and you end up doing more damage to your progress than you could have imagined. Instead of treating yourself to something bad to eat, you could challenge yourself to have something healthy in place of the treat and then feel twice as good later. Self-satisfaction is the biggest reward. Remember, it's still completely fine to treat yourself now and again to avoid binging. Have a cheat meal or a cheat day but fit it into your daily calorie limit and try to eat as nutritious as possible because nutrition is more important over calories.

CHAPTER 2:

Nutrition for Body Recomposition

While calorie counting is a touchy subject among many, some will argue that it is better that you don't do it. When your goals are to add muscle mass, you have to make sure that your body has the fuel it needs to increase and build the size of the muscle fibers. And if you start reducing your calorie intake, you will start losing fat. This helps to make you look more muscular, even though you aren't gaining new muscle.

You have to know what your true calorie needs are. You can't guess, estimate, or assume things about your habits. You need to use real data that is based upon what you do and who you are.

Since not everybody is the same, you can't give a baseline number for how many calories you need to consume. But lucky for you, there are a lot of online calculators that can do the math for you. Head over to bodybuilding.com and use their online calculator to figure out how many calories you should be aiming for during your different phases but as we are talking about body recomposition, let me show how to calculate your daily calorie intake later in this chapter.

If we provide our body with 3000 calories(through food and drinks) and expend 2000 calories in a day(whether from training, walking, sitting, or even being asleep), we have a net energy balance of +1000 calories. Those calories will be stored in our body as excess fat, muscle tissue or both. Most of the times is both when an individual follows a progressive overload training routine, though you should aim to maximize the muscle growth over the fat deposition.

In the case studied above, we have a positive net energy balance of +1000 calories. These are the conditions(caloric surplus) we should aim for when bulking, i.e. when aiming to build muscle. In other cases, where individuals would like to maintain their weight, their caloric intake should be maintenance calories, in which case their net energy balance is 0, by eating as many calories as they use up during each day.

Other than bulking and maintaining there are occasions when people would like to drop weight, loose fat. How is this one achieved? Yes, you guessed it right. And for achieving body recomposition, we need to be in negative energy balance by having a slight calorie deficit -10% from maintenance calories. This is accomplished by eating less, than your body uses to perform its various functions and activities.

What Is A Calorie Deficit?

The most important concept to understand before we begin, is a calorie deficit. In order to burn body fat, we need to create a calorie deficit. A calorie deficit is a state in which you burn more calories than you consume. For example, if you burn 2,500 calories per day and eat 2,250, you have created a deficit of 250(-10%) calories per day. A calorie deficit forces the body to use non-food sources of energy (typically body fat though the body can also burn muscle tissue for energy) to make up for the shortfall causing fat loss.

Setting A Calorie Deficit

A 3500 per week calorie deficit should be enough to help you decrease body fat whilst maintaining muscle. As you gain more experience, the rate at which you continue to build muscle will slowly decrease but your metabolic rate and body composition should be in a great place.

*Approximate calculations don't take into account muscle mass or training experience.

3500 Per Week Deficit= 1LB PER WEEK FAT LOSS

7000 Per Week Deficit= 2LB PER WEEK FAT LOSS

What Happens When We Over Deficit?

Most people go way too steep with their calorie deficit when trying to burn body fat and as a result they can't sustain their plan. As important as it is to create a calorie deficit for fat loss, there are many people who are very active that aren't consuming anywhere near enough calories and as a result their body composition remains the same. Sound familiar?

If you are very active and you are setting your weekly calorie targets too low, then over time you are essentially telling your body this is normality, making fat loss much tougher. The trick is to gradually deficit as your plan progresses over time.

Daily Caloric Intake for Men and Women

When preparing your meals, you will need to calculate their macronutrient breakdown and how many calories each meal contains. The included meal-plan provides this already if you choose to follow or pick days to eat from the 30-day meal plan. To benefit from this process, you need to know how much you need to eat each day. That's why daily caloric needs; also known as basal metabolic rate, is essential for keeping track of your daily macro intake. How to calculate your specific needs is explained below.

Why Mifflin St. Jeor Equation for Calculating BMR?

Among many formulas, the Mifflin-St Jeor Equation is considered the most accurate equation for calculating BMR with the exception that the Katch-McArdle Formula can be more accurate for people who are leaner and know their body fat percentage since we are talking about body recomposition, this formula is much more accurate for about 10-20% compared to other formulas.

Men: BMR = (9.99 x weight in kilograms) + (6.25 x height in centimeters) - 4.92 x age in years + 5.

Women: BMR = (9.99 x weight in kilograms) + (6.25 x height in centimeters) - (4.92 x age in years) - 161.

Multiply the BMR number with the activity factor that fits your lifestyle.

After you've estimated your BMR, you'll apply one among these physical activity factors to estimate your total energy needs.

Sedentary (little or no exercise, desk job).

BMR x 1.2

Lightly Active (light exercise/sports 3-5 days/week).

BMR x 1.3-1.4

Moderately Active (moderate exercise/sports 3-5 days/week).

BMR x 1.5-1.6

Very Active (hard exercise/sports 6-7 days per week).

BMR x 1.7-1.8

Extremely Active (very hard daily exercise/sports and physical job or 2/day training).

BMR x 1.9-2.0

Now, you have determined your maintenance calories. With that number calculate your calorie deficit, let's say 10% deficit.

I know, you are sick of doing maths, but it will be worth doing it.

Maintanance Calories x .10 = Deficit Calories. => Maintanance Calories – Deficit Calories = Daily Calorie Intake.

Now, we have to split our macronutrients within our daily calorie intake.

Calculating Your Daily Calorie Intake and Macronutrients Split

<u>Macros</u>

Macronutrients or "macros" is the name given to three groups of energy-dense nutrients which make up the most basic components of our diets: carbohydrates, fats, and proteins. In addition to acting as fuel for bodily energy, they facilitate many of our bodies' functions and are broken down by our digestive system for use in bodily structures. Each macronutrient provides us with the following number of calories:

1 g protein = 4 calories
1 g carb = 4 calories
1 g fat = 9 calories
Protein: 1 – 1.2 grams per pound of bodyweight per day.
Fats: 0.3 – 0.5 grams per pound of bodyweight per day.

Carbs: The remaining calories after setting protein and fat daily intake.

For Example:

Let's assume your BMR is 1600 and you workout with moderate intensity 3 times a week. So the physical activity level 1.5.

1600 x 1.5 = 2400

Now, 2400 is your Total Energy Expenditure (TEE) per day.

Now let's calculate your deficit calories (say, 10%).

2400 x .10 = 240

Minus 240 from TEE for daily intake calories.

2400 – 240 = 2160

Now, 2160 is your daily calorie needs. Now let's split your macronutrients.

Now, you weigh 150 lbs.

So, Protein = 1 gram per lb per day = 150 grams

150 x 4 = 600 calories (1 gram of protein = 4 calories)

Fats = 0.3 per lb per day = 45 grams

45 x 9 = 405 calories (1 gram of fat = 9 calories)

Carbs = Remaining calories = 2160 – 1005 (600 + 405) = 1155 calories

Carbs in gms = 1155 divide by 4 (1 gram of carb = 4 calories) = 288 grams

Tada, now you have your macronutrient split.

Lowering your carb and fat intakes will allow you to burn fat more efficiently. For people that pursue a fit lifestyle, a carb to protein to fat intake ratio of 50:25:25 is ideal. Once you have achieved your goals and wish to simply maintain your body weight, you need to focus on stabilizing your caloric intake with at least 15-20% of your calories coming from protein.

The following is a breakdown of how to achieve the 50:25:25 ratio on a 2000-calorie diet:

- 50% carbohydrates: 2000 x 50% = 1000 calories per day. To determine the grams needed, divide 1000 by 4 to get 250 grams of carbohydrates required on a daily basis.
- 25% protein: 2000 x 25% = 500 calories per day. Divide 500 calories by 4 to get 125 g of protein needed on a daily basis.
- 25% fat: 2000 x 25% = 500 calories per day. Divide 500 calories by 9 to get ~55.6 g of fat needed on a daily basis.

The Best Diet For Body Recomposition

When it comes to nutrition we are mainly concerned with the following: caloric intake, macronutrient split of those calories, water intake, fiber and micronutrients. We are going to deal with each one of them separately, but they are all of great importance, especially for an individual just like you and me who wants to keep his/her body healthy and keep it functioning at its optimal capacity.

If we provide our body with 3000 calories (through food and drinks) and expend 2000 calories in a day (whether from training, walking, sitting, or even being asleep), we have a net energy balance of +1000 calories. Those calories will be stored in our body as excess fat, muscle tissue or both. Most of the times is both when an individual follows a progressive overload training routine, though you should aim to maximize the muscle growth over the fat deposition.

Other than bulking and maintaining there are occasions when people would like to drop weight, loose fat. How is this one achieved? Yes, you guessed it right. By achieving a negative energy balance. This is accomplished by eating less, than your body uses to perform its various functions and activities.

Water

Water is important. Adult males are 60 percent water, while adult females' 70 percent. Muscles are about 70 percent water. For people like you and me who want to keep their body at its healthiest and maintain high levels of training performance, drinking enough water is essential.

So how much is enough water then? According to the Institute of Medicine women should consume 2.69 liters per day while men should take 3.69 liters per day. From these values we can subtract 20 percent, since we get water from food as well.

How much water you should drink varies from individual to individual according to the level of activity, environmental temperature and thus how much water is lost through transpiration(sweating).

Let's describe this in simple words so that everyone can visualize what is happening at the cellular level. These substances found in bottled water, attach to receptors (found on cells) whose primary function is to allow binding of hormones such as testosterone and estrogen. In this way these receptors are now blocked, and hormones are not able to bind. For this reason, these hormones cannot bring about their physiological function.

Keep in mind that you do not drink water once a day, or once a week. You drink lots of water, every single day. So small quantities of pollutants, bacteria and pharmaceuticals can accumulate in your body over time. Please stay away from that.

Fiber

You should have fiber in your diet. Before me giving the answer to how much of it we should be eating per day let me present to you all the positive effects fiber has on our health.

First of all, there are 2 forms of fiber. Soluble and insoluble fiber. The former (soluble fiber), stimulates the growth of healthy bacteria and fatty acids and fuels the colon Insoluble fiber is responsible for the renewal of the lining of the gastrointestinal tract, a process which is necessary for health

Common sources of soluble fiber include beans, peas, oats, plums, bananas, apples, broccoli, sweet potatoes, carrots and almonds. Insoluble fiber is found in brown rice, wheat bran, beans, peas, cauliflower, avocado and the skin of grapes, kiwis and tomatoes.

The time has to come to answer the question mentioned above. How much fiber should we take per day? According to the Institute of

Medicine, children and adults should consume 14g of fiber for every 1000 calories of food eaten

Protein

Protein is vital to the proper functioning of all living things. The basic molecules that make up proteins are amino acids, also known as "the building blocks of life".

Protein Requirements

During exercises, there is an increased protein breakdown and oxidation which is then followed by heightened muscle protein synthesis and further breakdown of proteins during recovery. So, for effective body recomposition, we need around 1 to 1.2 grams of protein per pound of body weight per day. The rise in the levels of circulating amino acids after one takes a protein-containing meal normally stimulates intramuscular protein synthesis in addition to slightly suppressing muscle breakdown of proteins.

Ingesting just carbohydrates into the body does not induce such increases in protein synthesis by the muscles. Furthermore, protein-containing meals have significant benefits to the immunity, muscle soreness as well as overall health as compared to carbohydrate-only meals.

Because of this, timing of protein content in meals is an important factor in recovery, muscle mass gain and maintenance.

The branched chain amino acids (BCAA) supplements; isoleucine, valine and leucine in a ratio of 1:1:2 have been specifically studied for their effects on muscle protein synthesis, performance and recovery. The oxidation of leucine supplements is significantly regulated during endurance exercises thus showing the necessity for increased intake of protein by athletes.

Research has suggested that the BCAA supplements do not affect performance significantly, but they attenuate exercise-induced muscle damages and also promote muscle protein synthesis. Plant proteins like sesame seeds, tofu, pumpkin seeds and sunflower seeds are great sources of BCAA supplements.

Amino acids compose many of the body's structures including nails, muscle, skin and hair. Some sources of vegan protein include tempeh, beans, quinoa, lentils, raw arugula, russet potatoes, raw collard greens, raw broccoli, raw spinach, boiled water chestnuts, boiled artichokes, boiled sweet corn and raw kale.

The table below shows the protein sources and their macronutrient breakdowns:

Food	Serving	Metric	Fats(g)	Carbs(g)	Fiber(g)	Protein(g)	Net Carbs(g)
Edamame	100g	100g	9	8.4	6	18.2	2.4
Lentils	100g	100g	0.4	20.1	7.9	9	12.2
White Beans	100g	100g	0.4	25.1	6.3	9.7	18.8
Cranberry Beans (Roman Beans)	100g	100g	0.5	24.5	8.6	9.3	15.9
Split Peas	100g	100g	0.4	21.1	8.3	8.3	12.8
Pinto Beans	100g	100g	0.7	26.2	9	9	17.2
Kidney Beans	100g	100g	0.5	22.8	6.4	8.7	16.4
Black Beans	100g	100g	0.5	23.7	8.7	8.9	15
Navy Beans	100g	100g	0.6	26.1	10.5	8.2	15.6
Lima Beans	100g	100g	0.3	23.6	5.4	6.8	18.2
Cornmeal (Grits)	100g	100g	3.6	76.9	7.3	8.1	69.6
Kamut	100g	100g	0.8	27.6	4.3	5.7	23.3
Teff, cooked	100g	100g	0.7	19.9	2.8	3.9	17.1
Quinoa	100g	100g	1.9	21.3	2.8	4.4	18.5
Couscous, cooked	1 oz.	86g	0.1	20	1.2	3.3	18.8
Oatmeal	100g	100g	1.5	12	1.7	2.5	10.3
Buckwheat Groats	100g	100g	0.6	19.9	2.7	3.4	17.2
Millet	100g	100g	1	23.7	1.3	3.5	22.4
Artichokes	100g	100g	0.2	10.5	5.4	10.5	5.1
Green Peas	100g	100g	0.2	15.6	5.5	5.4	10.1
Soybean Sprouts	½ cup	35g	2.3	3.3	0.4	4.6	3
Yellow Corn Sweet	100g	100g	1.4	18.7	2	3.3	16.7
Brussels Sprouts	½ cup	78g	0.4	5.5	2	2	3.5
Button Mushrooms	100g	100g	0.3	4	1.8	3.6	2.2
Broccoli	½ cup	78g	0.3	5.6	2.6	1.9	3
Guavas	100g	100g	1	14.3	5.4	2.6	8.9

Apricots	100g	100g	0.4	11.1	2	1.4	9.1
Kiwifruit	100g	100g	0.5	14.7	3	1.1	11.7
Blackberries	100g	100g	0.5	9.6	5.3	1.4	4.3
Oranges	100g	100g	0.1	11.8	2.4	0.9	9.4
Cantaloupe Melons	100g	100g	0.2	8.2	0.9	0.8	7.3
Hemp Seed	1 oz.	28g	13.8	2.5	1.1	9	1.3
Pumpkin Seeds	1 oz.	28g	13.9	4.2	1.8	8.5	2.3
Peanuts	1 oz.	28g	14.1	6	2.4	6	3.7
Pistachio Nuts	1 oz.	28g	13	8	2.9	6	5.1
Sunflower Seeds	1 oz.	28g	14.1	4.3	2.6	5.5	1.8
Pine Nuts	1 oz.	28g	19.4	3.7	1.1	3.9	2.7
Chickpeas	1 cup	164g	4.2	45	12.5	14.5	7.9
Amaranth	1 cup	28g	0.1	1.1	0	0.1	1.1

Amino acids are also involved in many of the body's chemical reactions, as they are the basic components of enzymatic structures and other chemical molecules. This ultimately means that they regulate mood, growth, and tissue repair, as they control the buildup and breakdown of complex molecules.

A couple of exceptional plant foods are soy and quinoa, which contain a great balance of amino acids. Soy contains all nine essential amino acids, making it a complete protein source.

Can't I get fat from consuming too much protein?

Theoretically, you can put fat on by supercharging one of the macronutrients, but among the 3, the protein is the most difficult for the body to convert into body fat and for this reason, more lean protein can be consumed without fear of gaining weight compared to overeating with carbohydrates or fats. Excess protein can be converted into carbohydrates in the body, which can then be converted to fat, but this conversion is expensive and is actually fueled by burning fat. Often, excessive cravings for carbohydrates can come from a lack of amino acids in the brain and the bloodstream that leaves proteins, and these cravings can often be alleviated with adequate consumption of proteins. So be sure to get enough protein often!

Protein before training

But not all sources of protein are created equal. Different sources of protein have different absorption rates. Fast digesting protein like whey, will spike your plasma(blood) amino acid levels sooner than other sources of protein like casein which is slower digesting/acting.

A spike in amino acid levels will induce anabolic conditions. Anabolism is the biological process which joins small molecules(micro-molecules) to form a more complex, bigger molecule(macromolecules). Just like building a tall wall. We use many small bricks to build something bigger. In this analogy, the bricks are paralleled to amino acids and the wall, are the new muscle fibers.

When you are training, you are causing micro-damage, also known as micro-tears to your muscle fibers This is a process called catabolism; the biological mechanism exactly opposite to anabolism. It is responsible to break bigger molecules(macromolecules) down into smaller/simpler ones(micro-molecules); i.e. breaking down muscular protein (also known as proteolysis).

As of the timing of your pre-workout protein intake, I want you to be asking yourself the following question: ''what will my amino acid levels be at the time of training?''. When did I last eat protein, and how many grams of protein did I eat?

If on the other hand you ate 200g of chicken breast (62g of protein) 2 hours before training, then there is no need for any extra protein. Just because you will be hitting the weights, does not mean you should always have a shaker of dissolved protein powder, or BCAAs next to you all the time. It really comes down to when you last ate protein and how many grams of it.

Protein after training

During training, proteolysis and more specifically muscle proteolysis, is constant, however it increases even more after training. When the rate of breaking down muscle protein is higher than the rate of muscle protein synthesis, it results in muscle loss.

So, for this reason, I would suggest you eat a post workout meal maximum 3 hours after training. The sooner the better though. In case you will not be able to get a post workout meal after training, you should use a whey protein supplement, though I don't think most people are that busy.

Eating protein 3 hours after training is better than 5 hours. Eating protein 1 hour after training is better than 3 hours. But that doesn't mean you have to take protein right after training.

With that being said, which means "anabolic window" is indeed not true. For those of you unfamiliar with this term, it means that you should be eating protein as soon as you are done with lifting weights. Having your protein intake any time within three hours after training would do the work but not necessarily right after your workout. It doesn't matter when you take your protein within those three hours post workout.

According to research, individuals who ate protein within the first three hours after training showed 30 to 100 percent more protein synthesis than individuals who ate protein later than five hours after their training session.

Keep in mind, small positive changes add up over time when they occur systematically. I would suggest you eat a minimum of 25 - 40grams of protein anytime within the three hours post workout. With this we are turning off the switch for negative net muscle protein balance(catabolism) and turning it on for a positive net muscle protein balance(anabolism), without remaining into a catabolic state for an extended period of time. Stay anabolic my friend. Stay anabolic!

Fats

Over the past three decades, it has been drilled into our minds that fats are bad. Period. However, the truth of the matter is that the body needs fats. For one, we need fat to absorb certain fat-soluble vitamins like A, D, E and K. Without fat, the body is not able to absorb those much-needed vitamins. Additionally, we need fat for healthy skin and hair as well as a protective insulator.

Your body is unable to produce essential fatty acids, so it is critical that you consume good fat sources. These essential fats help with numerous body processes like regulating blood pressure, protecting organs and brain development functions.

Consuming unsaturated fats is your best bet. Unsaturated fats are in a liquid state and generally come from plant sources. Saturated fats are solid and generally come from animal sources. Trans fats are a third major fat. These fats are often produced by companies trying to increase the shelf life of their products. Trans fats are unsaturated fats that are turned into saturated fats by hydrogenizing the unsaturated fat. Needless to say, trans fats are super bad and should be avoided.

Plant-based oils are a great vegan source of unsaturated fats. Butters like cocoa butter and coconut cream are also great sources of healthy vegan fats. There have been studies stating coconut oil is "overrated" as it only temporarily aids your body's nutritional levels. In fact, while coconut oil may claim to decrease LDL levels (your "bad" cholesterol levels) it actually eventually adds to your LDL levels in the long run. As a result, while many recipes lean towards the use of coconut oil, remember that any oil of your choice works just as well. These include sunflower oil, flax seed oil and olive oil, which give your body a well-balanced array of fats. Okay, then how much of fat do we need for effective body recomposition? We need around 0.3 to 0.5 grams of fat per pound of body weight per day.

Fats before training

Fats are the least important of all macronutrients when it comes to pre-workout nutrition. Research done in 2004 by Deakin University, has shown that fats do not induce any improvement in training performance. Carbohydrates and protein are all you need before a training session.

If you would like to eat something that contains fat in it along with carbohydrates, so be it, but focus on the two aforementioned macronutrients. 40g of protein and 40+g of carbohydrates. You are all prepared now to head to the gym and have an amazing session.

Fats after training

You should not worry about fats. Consider them as something complimentary. Make sure to get the 2 macronutrients mentioned above at the right amounts and the right time. Anyways, there will be some fats in the food you eat in order to get the desired carbohydrates and protein, but again, fats have no significant effect on the muscle breakdown-muscle synthesis balance.

Omega 3-6-9

Fatty acids are vital for your body's functions, from your respiratory and circulatory systems to your brain and other vital organs. Ultimately, while the body does produce fatty acids such as the Omega-9 fatty acid on its, there are two essential fatty acids (EFAs) it cannot produce: Omega-3 and Omega-6.

The Omega-3 fatty acid is responsible for aiding in brain function as well as preventing cardiovascular disease. This fatty acid prevents asthma, certain cancers, arthritis, high cholesterol, blood pressure and so on. Many say that our dosage of Omega-3 can be satisfied by consuming fatty fish such as salmon however, it's a great misconception that vegans lack this vital nutrient due to not consuming fatty-flesh foods. While Omega-3 is most popularly taken from fish, it has a plethora of vegan sources as well, including green vegetables, chia seed oil, flaxseed oils, raw walnuts and hempseed oil to name a few!

The Omega-6 fatty acid is responsible for many of the benefits mentioned above when consumed with Omega-3. Omega-6 can be found in seeds, nuts, green veggies and oils, such as olive oil. The trick is to consume the right levels of these nutrients; you should be consuming double the amount of Omega-6 fatty acid as the Omega-3 or the benefits of these EFAs may actually be cancelled. The world has become victim to fast food and frozen pre-made dishes that have dangerously high amounts of Omega-6; but following a whole foods based diet can ensure your health as you get balanced amounts of each and every nutrient.

The Omega-9 fatty acid is a non-essential fatty acid which the body can produce. Although the body will only produce this fatty acid once there are appropriate levels of both Omega-3 and Omega-6, thus making it dependent on the consumption of the two fatty acids the body cannot produce. If you do not have appropriate amounts of Omega-3 and Omega-6, then you can get additional Omega-9 from your diet (since your body wouldn't be producing it in this case). Omega-9 can be found naturally in avocados, nuts, chia seed oil and olive oil.

Carbs

Carbohydrates are the human body's main energy source and are classed into two groups: simple and complex. Simple carbohydrates are low in nutrients and fiber and are easily broken down into glucose to generate energy. Complex carbohydrates consist of long chains of monosaccharides which take longer to be broken down. Unlike simple carbohydrates, they contain fiber (which keeps you satiated longer after a meal), minerals and vitamins. Complex carbohydrate plant sources include whole grains, lentils, legumes, beans, sweet potatoes and cruciferous.

The Glycemic Index (GI) is a scale used to rank carbohydrates according to the rise of glucose levels in the blood after consumption. High GI carbs release glucose into the blood very rapidly, commonly known as blood sugar spikes. These blood sugar spikes caused by simple carbs should be avoided and can eventually be the cause of diabetes type 2. Complex carbs release glucose slowly because of a low GI (less than 55). Complex carbs are helpful in keeping a stable blood sugar level and should be a staple in your diet. source of vitamin D is, of course, sunlight, if you live in a predominantly cloudy region of the world, it's a good idea to supplement. Now, how many carbs should I consume per day? Well, once your protein and fats intake are set for the day, the remaining calories from your total calories are for carbs.

Carbohydrates before training

Before your training session you should provide your body with fuel. Your main go to in order to increase performance, are simple carbohydrates (fast digesting and absorbing).

When should you eat this pre-workout carbohydrates? As a general rule of thumb, you should give your system 15-30 minutes to digest these carbohydrates, though this may vary slightly from individual to individual according to their metabolism, the rate at which biological processes take place in one's body.

As of the carbohydrate supplements, e.g. dextrose, I would suggest you stay away from that. They are just over-priced, and you can simply take all the desired carbohydrates from food. Much more enjoyable, right?

A question that may come up is: ''Do carbohydrates affect muscle growth?''. In answer to that, yes, carbohydrates do affect muscle growth, indirectly. Carbohydrates are not made up of amino acids, as we have seen in the case of protein, but by sugars.

Sugars are not used as monomers in muscle tissue formation, but are used to fuel your workouts, resulting in more repetitions being dialed in, in every set, accumulating more workload in each session. So, carbohydrates are important. We will discuss about the role of insulin in the section of post-workout protein ingestion.

Carbohydrates after training

You need carbohydrates after training. Carbohydrates are broken down into simple sugars, more specifically glucose. An increase of glucose levels in the blood causes your pancreas to secrete insulin.

According to a research, you can have the desired insulin spike and its effects by eating just protein, via a process known as gluconeogenesis. In this process glucogenic amino acids (from protein) are converted to sugars.

During training, muscular glycogen (a polymer of sugars in the muscles), is broken down to glucose to provide the fuel for energy production. Soon, these glycogen stores get depleted. When an individual train with depleted glycogen stores, muscle breakdown is accelerated. We definitely not want that. Also, fully restored glycogen stores contribute to better performance in sports..

Micronutrients

Micronutrients include vitamins and minerals. Antioxidants and phytochemicals are also categorized as micronutrients, but we will not deal with these here.

Vitamins are organic compounds that we either not make enough in our body, or not make at all, therefore we need to get them from food. There are 13 different vitamins. Their functions include enzyme activation, collagen production, assisting in the digestion of macronutrients (better absorption of protein), blood sugar regulation, among others.

Minerals are elements (Calcium, Phosphorus, Magnesium, Iron, Zinc, Iodine etc.). We need some of them in major amounts while others in trace amounts. Their functions include water balance, blood cell production, cognitive benefits, blood sugar regulation, to name a few.

So, how do we provide our system with these micronutrients? By choosing a diet consisting of a variety of nutrient-dense foods such as avocados, Brussels sprouts, baked potatoes, sweet potatoes, berries, eggs, lentils, peas, salmon, lean beef, chicken, turkey, shrimps, tuna among others.

Daily Needs of Micronutrients

Micronutrient	Recommended Dietary Allowance
Calcium	1200 mg
Phosphorus	700 mg
Magnesium	400 mg for men and 310 mg for women
Potassium	4700 mg
Sodium	1500 mg
Chloride	2300 mg
Iron	8 mg for men and 18 mg for women
Zinc	11 mg for men, 8 mg for women
Copper	900 µg
Iodine	150 µg
Manganese	2.3 mg for men, 1.8 mg for women
Vitamin A	900 µg for men, 700 µg for women
Vitamin D	15 µg
Vitamin E	15 mg
Vitamin K	120 µg for men, 90 µg for women
Vitamin C	90 mg for men, 75 mg for women
Thiamine (B1)	1.2 mg for men, 1.1 mg for women
Riboflavin (B2)	1.3 mg for men, 1.1 mg for women
Niacin (B3)	16 mg for men, 14 mg for women
Pantothenic acid (B5)	1.3 mg
Pyridoxine (B6)	1.3 mg
Biotin (B7)	30 µg
Folic acid (B9)	400 µg
Cobalamin/Vitamin B12	2.4 µg

Micronutrient Intake

Micronutrients (vitamins and minerals) play important roles in most of the body's functions. Vitamins fall into two categories: water-soluble vitamins (C and B complex) and fat-soluble vitamins (A, D, E & K) – see chart below. Water-soluble vitamins are held in the body for up to three days and therefore need to be replaced regularly throughout the diet while fat-soluble vitamins can be stored in the liver for up to a year.

On a vegan diet, particular attention needs to be paid to vitamin D, calcium and vitamin B12. Vitamin B12, which plays a vital role in the procession of oxygen-carrying red blood cells, is predominantly found in animal products. Based on recommendations, an adult should consume 2.4mcg of vitamin B12 per day. On a vegan diet it would be wise to supplement and be vigilant about consuming foods such as B12-fortified cereals. Please talk to your nutritionist or dietician about the best way to supplement.

Good plant sources of calcium include leafy greens such as collards and kale, as well as plant-based milk alternatives like soy, almond, rice, or hemp milk. Vitamin D sources include portobello and shiitake mushrooms, as well as fortified milk alternatives. Though the best source of vitamin D is, of course, sunlight, if you live in a predominantly cloudy region of the world, it's a good idea to supplement.

Ideally, eat between 4-6 meals a day

When you eat frequent and smaller meals, the body is better able to use all the nutrients without worrying about gaining fat. Hunger and cravings are better stabilized, and energy levels are more stable. Frequent meals have a helpful effect on the regulation of appetite and prevent significant peaks and troughs in blood sugar, which contributes to binge eating. Since a calorie is actually a unit of heat, if we ingest calories that help us burn more calories during digestion, while eating quite frequently, we gain a metabolic benefit. You can do this by eating regular meals with each protein-containing meal.

Snacks - Focus on fibrous vegetables and protein Snacks can be a very good thing, but most individuals make the mistake of not eating often enough. Therefore, when they take a snack, they are hungry for sweets, sugars, and other easily digestible carbohydrates. When carbohydrates like these are consumed alone, the effect on blood sugar and insulin is dramatic. In general, when you eat a snack or meal containing carbohydrates, energy is provided faster than the body can burn it, which in turn lead to fat buildup.

Muscles need amino acids for growth and carbohydrate storage for energy, so there are times when high levels of insulin can improve muscle storage, which is a good thing. Timing and food is everything! The times when it is best to have high insulin levels, or when the body is most able to use insulin to direct nutrients to muscles and not to fat, is when sensitivity to l muscle insulin is the highest; When they are in an exhausted or semi-exhausted state. At these times, less insulin is needed for muscles to absorb nutrients. These deadlines are generally: **Breakfast** (We didn't eat all night, so our glycogen levels are low) **After training** - Within 3 hours after a period of exercise. Exercise, especially higher intensity exercise, makes muscle cells much more sensitive to insulin, so insulin directs nutrients to muscle cells rather than fat cells at this point.

For optimal fat loss, at any other time, it is best to avoid high insulin levels because the muscles are less receptive and a rise in insulin levels by eating very high sugar and carbohydrate-rich meals. will cause more nutrients to be stored in fat rather than muscle.

You can still take in carbohydrates throughout the day and at other times, but you should focus on "complex carbohydrates" rather than sugars, which break down more slowly and stimulate low to moderate insulin release.

Eating Healthy and Losing Weight

Through preparing and storing meals, you will also be able to learn how to control your portion intake, since you will be using containers made up of compartments intended for the separation of meal components into the desired portions. When dividing portions, there are a number of aspects to consider, including calorie count and macronutrient proportions. Taking in a lower number of calories will help you shed some weight. The number of daily calories required in order to lose weight are shown in the percentage-based caloric deficit table below. These will not be empty calories as the vegan meals you prepare will be packed with nutrition to increase performance, brainpower and general health.

Be sure to note the nutritional information of each meal on the storage containers you use, as well as the weight of the portion. Once your containers are labeled, you can estimate the daily number of calories and macros you will be taking in. To make it easy sticking to the caloric deficit required to achieve your goals. Calculating your daily caloric needs will be explained in the subchapter "Counting calories".

Daily Caloric Needs	20% Caloric Deficit
1600 calories	320 calories below the maintenance level (1280 calories on a daily basis)
1800 calories	360 calories below the maintenance level (1440 calories on a daily basis)
2000 calories	400 calories below the maintenance level (1600 calories on a daily basis)
2500 calories	500 calories below the maintenance level (2000 calories on a daily basis)
3000 calories	600 calories below the maintenance level (2400 calories on a daily basis)
4000 calories	800 calories below the maintenance level (3200 calories on a daily basis)

The Best Diet

With that being said, the next question that may arise is: "Which one is the best diet to follow?". Paleo, intermittent fasting, ketogenic diet and the list goes on. The answer to that is simple. The diet which you can follow. A diet which is sustainable and enjoyable. One that contains nutritious healthy, micronutrient rich foods that you look forward to eating and also contains some of your favorite processed, less healthy foods (kept to a minimum).

Your major concern though, should be to make sure that those junk foods, sweets, or whatever else your tooth craves, actually fit into your macronutrient split we mentioned above for your own specific goal.

There are lots of different calorie tracking applications, you can download, which will make it easy for you to know how many calories, protein, carbohydrates, fats etc are contained in anything that you eat. An application that I used for a couple of years in the past is called

MyFitnessPal.

If you do not like the idea of tracking calories after every meal that you eat, you can get a nutritionist/dietitian to form a nutrition plan for you. In this way you know exactly how much and what to eat and can prepare your meals for the day in advance and just eat them whenever it is time to eat or whenever you feel hungry.

As of the rest meals of the day, you can eat them whenever you want. The more equally spaced the better though. Their timing is minimally important when compared to that of the pre-workout and post-workout meals.

Lack of vitamins and minerals will severely affect your health other than your performance in the gym. In addition to that, the low-quality protein found in their patties, won't be the best source of amino acids for muscle tissue maintenance, repair and synthesis. So make sure you get high quality protein and sufficient vitamin rich foods in your diet.

CHAPTER 3:

Training for Body Recomposition

There is no doubt about it: Body recomposition is an intimidating task. When starting your body recomposition journey, you need to start out on the right foot to prevent burning out in the long term. Many aspiring people begin with regimens that are too intense for what they're used to, and the result is failure and burnout.

Below is a great program that uses simple techniques for body recomposition to establish that important muscle mass and core strength. It consists the number of days you will have to train, and their gap will vary based on your schedule.

It's common for people seeking weight loss to drastically change their workout program from a lower rep, heavier weight sort of training to at least one of lighter weight, higher reps. this is often usually done under the misunderstanding that higher reps are better for fat loss and cause better muscle "toning." or they think we should always just start doing more cardio – which isn't the case. We first should be prioritizing training that builds muscle mass (yes, even while cutting).

But, performing tons of high rep, light weight workouts does little for building muscle and next to zilch for increasing strength -- both of which should be what you're trying to do when recomping.

The only way to improve strength and build muscle while recomping is performing multi-joint exercises (e.g. squats, bench, deadlift, rows, etc) with heavy weight. The three main components to training for muscle mass and strength are Volume, Intensity, and Frequency.

Training frequency, is what most people do not take it seriously, they tend to workout one muscle per week and that isn't enough. Training each muscle group at least 2 -3 times per week is optimal for building muscle and strength. So, now let us look into the concept of Strength Training.

Strength Training

Strength training involves lifting weights with the goal of accelerating your whole-body strength the maximum amount of weight as possible.

- Emphasizes sets of lower reps (4 to 6) over sets of higher reps (6 to 15+).
- Compound movements which involves multiple joints and muscle groups are performed and such exercises are the Deadlift, Squat, Bench Press, Lunges, Pullups, Military Press, Rows etc..
- Prioritizes weight over reps
- The rest period is long enough to recover before the next set.

How to Design a Strength Training Program

There are few principles we need to follow for building an effective strength training program:

Progressive overload is must

If you are lifting the same weight for 6 months then you probably wouldn't have built any muscle and strength.

You have to progressively overload the weight you lift, which means you have to increase the weight every other week.

If you do not add weight to the bar, then it is not strength training at all, it is just bunch of random exercises.

Training frequency is important

It is recommended to hit each muscle group at least 2 – 3 times per week because that is what various number of studies have proved and it actually makes sense because hitting only one muscle group a week is only going to trigger that particular muscle group and it has to wait for another one week to get trained which leads to less muscle growth and strength. If you are hitting each muscle group multiple times a week after giving sufficient rest period to recover and that is when you are building muscle and strength optimally.

And this is how you can achieve this:

- 3 Day Split
- 4 Day Split
- 5 Day Split

Enough rest period between sets

Studies shows that folks who rest longer between sets are actually capable to gain more strength and muscle than people who rest less.

How long do you have to rest?

You should rest as long as you would like to feel fully prepared for the subsequent set. This usually works bent around three minutes between your heaviest sets and two minutes between your lighter sets or smaller exercises, although on some days you'll need even longer than this.

The bottom line is that if you would like to put on muscle and strength, you should lift heavy weights, no other go. And if you would like to lift heavy weights, you would like to rest long enough between sets to handle heavier and heavier weights.

Know your workout intensity

In order to know this, you have to know your 1 rep max for each exercise, especially for the big three (Deadlift, Squat and Bench Press).

What is one-rep max?

A one-rep max (1RM) is that the maximum amount of weight you'll lift for one repetition of a given exercise through a full range of motion with proper technique.

Knowing your 1RM helps you maintain optimal workout intensity (and thereby achieve optimal results).

It allows you to work hard enough to urge the utmost muscle-building stimulus out of each workout, without training so hard that you simply increase the danger of getting injured or running into symptoms associated with overtraining.

Most of the time, your weights are supported a percentage of your 1RM. for instance , studies suggest to use a weight that's 80% of your one-rep max for many of your sets.

Now, the sole 100%-accurate method to determine how much weight you'll lift for one rep is to truly do it, but that comes at a price .

A true 1RM attempt is time-consuming, risky, and exhausting.

It's unnecessary, unless you're preparing for a powerlifting competition.

This is why most of the people rarely do true 1RM tests. Instead, they use equations to predict their 1RM based on how many reps they will get with a lighter weight.

For example, if you deadlift a weight that you can do 5 reps before reaching failure, you'll then put the load and reps into a calculator to estimate your 1RM.

These equations can predict your 1RM very accurately, especially if you employ a weight that permits you to urge 10 or fewer reps.

To use one among these equations, you initially got to test your "rep max," which is is that the amount of weight you'll lift for a given number of reps.

For example, if you can deadlift 200 pounds for 3 reps, that's your "3-rep max" (3RM).

You'll get an accurate estimate of your 1RM just by reviewing your training logs from the past few weeks, finding the foremost weight you lifted for an exercise and for how many reps, then putting those numbers into the 1RM calculator which is available online. I use Legionathletics 1 RM calculator.

So, how much should you lift?

It is recommended to lift 80% – 85% of your 1RM.

Building The Training Program

A strength training program has the following principles:

1. Train multiple muscle groups per day.
2. Perform 4 to 6 reps for compound exercises and 8 to 12 reps for isolation exercises.
3. Perform 9 to 12 heavy sets per workout.
4. Warmup sets are must for compound exercises.
5. Perform large muscle groups (compound exercises) first.
6. Rest 2 – 3 minutes between sets.
7. Train about a hour per workout.
8. Static stretch the muscles after the workout.
9. Give at least 24 hour recovery period between workouts.
10. Train each muscle group 2 or 3 times a week.

Let us see the split workout routines I have used in my past.

NOTE: You can build your own strength training program based on the principles we have learnt from this chapter.

3 Day Full Body Workout Routine

Workout A - Monday

Warmup sets
3 – 4 sets of 80 – 85 percent of 1RM for 4 – 6 reps
Squats
Bench Press
Lat Pulldowns
Military Press
3 sets of 70 – 75 percent of 1RM for 8 – 12 reps
Leg Curls
Bicep Curls

Face Pulls

Workout B - Wednesday

Warmup sets
3 – 4 sets of 80 – 85 percent of 1RM for 4 – 6 reps
Romanian Deadlifts
Inclined Dumbell Press
Seated Cable Rows
Leg Press
3 sets of 70 – 75 percent of 1RM for 8 – 12 reps
Lateral Raises
Tricep Pushdowns

Standing Calf Raises

Workout C – Friday

Warmup sets
3 – 4 sets of 80 – 85 percent of 1RM for 4 – 6 reps
Barbell Hip Thrusts
Bodyweight/Weighted Chest Dips
Bodyweight/Weighted Pullups
Dumbell Lunges

3 sets of 70 – 75 percent of 1RM for 8 – 12 reps
Shoulder Shrugs
Triceps Extensions

Preacher Curls

4 Day Upper/Lower Workout Routine

Upper – Monday

Warmup sets
3 – 4 sets of 80 – 85 percent of 1RM for 4 – 6 reps
Bench Press
Lat Pulldown
Incline Bench Press
Seated Rows
Military Press
3 sets of 70 – 75 percent of 1RM for 8 – 12 reps
Lateral Raises
Dumbell Tricep Extension

Dumbell Bicep Curls

Lower - Tuesday

Warmup sets
3 – 4 sets of 80 – 85 percent of 1RM for 4 – 6 reps
Deadlift
Back Squat
Leg Press
Dumbell Lunges
3 sets of 70 – 75 percent of 1RM for 8 – 12 reps
Leg Extension
Leg Curls

Standing Calf Raises

Upper – Thursday

Warmup sets
3 – 4 sets of 80 – 85 percent of 1RM for 4 – 6 reps
Barbell Rows
Decline Dumbell Press
Bodyweight/Weighted Inverted Rows
Incline Dumbell Press
Dumbell Shoulder Press
3 sets of 70 – 75 percent of 1RM for 8 – 12 reps
Bent Over Raises
Tricep Pushdown

Barbell Curls

Lower - Friday

Warmup sets
3 – 4 sets of 80 – 85 percent of 1RM for 4 – 6 reps
Romaninan Deadlift
Front Squat
Hip Thrusts
Dumbell Lunges
3 sets of 70 – 75 percent of 1RM for 8 – 12 reps
Leg Extension
Leg Curls

Standing Calf Raises

5 Day Push/Pull/Legs Workout Routine

Lower Body Week

Legs A - Monday

Warmup sets
3 – 4 sets of 80 – 85 percent of 1RM for 4 – 6 reps
Front Squat
Dealift
Leg Press

3 sets of 70 – 75 percent of 1RM for 8 – 12 reps

Standing Calf Raises

Push A – Tuesday

Warmup sets
3 – 4 sets of 80 – 85 percent of 1RM for 4 – 6 reps
Bench Press
Standing Military Press
Weighted Dips
3 sets of 70 – 75 percent of 1RM for 8 – 12 reps

Lateral Raises

Pull A – Wednesday

Warmup sets
3 – 4 sets of 80 – 85 percent of 1RM for 4 – 6 reps
Barbell Rows
Pullups (As many as possible)
Cable Rows
3 sets of 70 – 75 percent of 1RM for 8 – 12 reps

One Arm Dumbell Row

Legs B – Thursday

Warmup sets
3 – 4 sets of 80 – 85 percent of 1RM for 4 – 6 reps
Back Squat
Romanian Deadlift
Hip Thrusts
3 sets of 70 – 75 percent of 1RM for 8 – 12 reps

Standing Calf Raises

Push B – Friday

Warmup sets

3 – 4 sets of 80 – 85 percent of 1RM for 4 – 6 reps
Incline Bench Press
Seated Military Press
Close Grip Bench Press
3 sets of 70 – 75 percent of 1RM for 8 – 12 reps

Lateral Raises

Upper Body Week

Push A – Monday

Warmup sets
3 – 4 sets of 80 – 85 percent of 1RM for 4 – 6 reps
Bench Press
Standing Military Press
Weighted Dips
3 sets of 70 – 75 percent of 1RM for 8 – 12 reps

Lateral Raises

Pull A – Tuesday

Warmup sets
3 – 4 sets of 80 – 85 percent of 1RM for 4 – 6 reps
Barbell Rows
Pullups (As many as possible)
Cable Rows
3 sets of 70 – 75 percent of 1RM for 8 – 12 reps

One Arm Dumbell Row

Legs A - Wednesday

Warmup sets
3 – 4 sets of 80 – 85 percent of 1RM for 4 – 6 reps
Front Squat
Dealift
Leg Press

3 sets of 70 – 75 percent of 1RM for 8 – 12 reps

Standing Calf Raises

Push B – Thursday

Warmup sets
3 – 4 sets of 80 – 85 percent of 1RM for 4 – 6 reps
Incline Bench Press
Seated Military Press
Close Grip Bench Press
3 sets of 70 – 75 percent of 1RM for 8 – 12 reps

Lateral Raises

Pull B – Friday

Warmup sets
3 – 4 sets of 80 – 85 percent of 1RM for 4 – 6 reps
Barbell Rows
Chinups (As many as possible)
Lat Pulldowns
3 sets of 70 – 75 percent of 1RM for 8 – 12 reps

One Arm Dumbell Row

Here you have got strength training programs for all split routines. Now, let me tell you to whom does each workout program is suitable.

If you are just starting out to workout, a complete beginner, I would suggest you to go with the 3 day split.

If you have already worked out in the past and you are an intermediate lifter, but have sitting idle for the past few months, then go with 4 day split routine.

If you are already training and you have hit a plateau and also you are an advanced lifter, then go with 5 day split routine.

Now, let's talk about cardio.

HIIT Cardio

So, what is HIIT?
High Intensity Interval Training.

But what is it dude?

High-Intensity Interval Training is sort of cardiovascular activity that's done in a short period of time but long on calorie burn. It provides the simplest bang for your buck in terms of getting the increased energy expenditure of cardio without having to eat away muscle tissue or waste hours of your day on the treadmill or elliptical machine.

HIIT is performed by alternating periods of all-out effort and periods of low-to-moderate intensity effort, usually at a work-to-rest ratio of 1:2 or 1:3, counting on your level of conditioning.

Lot of studies have shown that interval training burns more fat than steady-state cardio (LISS).

In addition to greater fat loss, HIIT also comes with sort of other benefits, including:

- Increased resting rate for up to 24 hours post exercise.
- Increased levels of skeletal muscle fat oxidation (fat burning)
- Greater insulin sensitivity in skeletal muscle
- Post-workout appetite suppression
- Statistically significant spikes in anabolic hormones and fat-burning catecholamines like adrenaline and noradrenaline

But that's not all.

HIIT is better when it involves preserving muscle and strength compared to LISS cardio.

But, when should I do HIIT cardio in a week?
I would recommend around 2 – 3 sessions per week.

And those sessions would fit in your schedule like below:

If you are following the 3 day split, do the HIIT cardio on Tuesday and Saturday.

If you are following the 4 day split, do the HIIT cardio on Wednesday and Saturday

If you are following the 5 day split, do the HIIT cardio on your push and pull days after your workout.

And how many minutes should each session be?

A session should last from 20 to 30 minutes maximum and not more than that because you might get injured.

And this is how it should be:

Start your HIIT session with a low-to-moderate intensity 5-minute warm up and when your warm up is complete, start off with your first "sprint" (max effort period) for 20 to 30 seconds. After the max effort period, the transition to your "active recovery" interval for 60 seconds moving at a low-to-moderate intensity.

Repeat this on-off cycle for 20-30 minutes then end your workout with another 5 minute cooldown.

Important Considerations

Whatever regimen you choose, it is important to first warmup and dynamic stretch no matter what before you start your workout to get your blood flowing so your body is in optimal shape during the workout. Also, each workout should be accompanied by around 20 minutes of cardiovascular workouts to further prevent injury.

Keep it simple at first. Don't go all out on the isolation exercises and concentrate on fusion multi-joint workouts. A great starter routine needs to be continued for the first 8 to 10 weeks in order to allow sufficient time for the body to accommodate to the exercises and grow a solid foundation of strength and mass. Once that is achieved, workouts can be switched, and the format arranged slightly.

Combine these workouts with our diet and hydration plan to feel great, have energy you never had before, and make the best gains of your life!

For maximum results stick previously set assumptions.

- Set a Goal
- Calculate Caloric Needs
- Train According to the Established Workout Plan
- Stick to Diet Assumptions, and Count Calories
- Track the Effects

CHAPTER 4:

Sleep For Body Recomposition

Sleep is that the foundation of a proper muscle building routine. It gives us the drive to challenge ourselves within the gym, the appetite to eat an enormous muscle-building diet, and therefore the willpower to implement new habits. Except for the sake of giving sleep the credit it deserves, let's not forgot that it improves our willpower, motivation, compliance, exertion, and every one of the super important secondary benefits. Here's how sleep can directly increase muscle hypertrophy and strength gains:

- Increased testosterone.
- Increased Insulin-like Growth Factor (IGF-1)
- Less Cortisol
- Less Inflammation
- Increased Muscle Growth

If we give sleep high priority in our lives, it won't just improve our muscle growth, it'll improve everything.

Before getting into the how part, let me explain the why part first.

Why does lack of sleep make us more likely to incur injury?

Sleep allows the body to regenerate damaged cells–cells damaged during training and just life generally .

Halson and Juliff (2017) write that sleep features a role in "performance, illness, injury, metabolism, cognition, memory, learning, and mood... (and that) slow wave sleep provides a restorative function...by repairing processes and restoring energy."

Without adequate sleep, recovery, cognition and mood will all be affected, and performance are going to be affected negatively.

When we don't give our bodies enough opportunity for self repair and regeneration, we start to interrupt down little by little, until small amounts of injury accumulate into major injuries.

And once we don't sleep enough to get over hard training and our busy lives, we are more likely to urge run down and sick too. Sleep repairs our immune systems–making us ready to defend against foreign invaders and bacteria. once we don't sleep enough, we find yourself getting sick more often.

More time spent sick means less time spent within the gym, or on the sector , making improvements and getting better–limiting our progress over the long run also .

There is evidence that not getting enough sleep can compromise our basic health and longevity.

Inadequate sleep can cause poor mood and depression, high vital sign , weight gain, heart condition , and may even affect our lifespan.

In contrast, extending the time we spend sleeping can have profound impacts on our performance, health and longevity. people that get enough sleep tend to measure longer than people who don't.

Why is Adequate Sleep so Crucial for Muscle Building?

Sleep is incredibly important for muscle building, not just by improving our performance and helping us have more focused, productive sessions, but also by improving our muscle building mass.

Sleep allows our bodies to enter a particularly anabolic (muscle building) period, where human growth hormone , testosterone and melatonin are all elevated. These hormones help us heal micro-damage to the muscle cells and also build new muscle tissue. These hormones also help us burn body fat.

Sleep really is our greatest friend for improving body composition, our fat free mass, and reducing our total fat mass.

Dattilo et. Al (2011) actually wrote that the absence of sleep results in reductions in natural levels of anabolic hormones like testosterone and insulin-like growth factor 1, resulting in more muscle protein breakdown (more muscle loss) and fewer muscle protein synthesis (muscle gain).

Dattilo also hypothesizes that inadequate sleep hinders the recovery or certain injuries and exacerbated muscle protein breakdown in individuals with chronic illness.

Serious Training Puts Strain on Muscles and Connective tissue

Strength training does stress and strain the whole body—including the muscles, bones, connective tissue , hormonal and endocrine systems.

The more strenuous the training, the more of these systems are going to be affected.

With adequate rest, our body can adapt to the stressors—and the muscles, bones, connective tissues and joints, and endocrine systems will all respond positively.

Without adequate sleep, our bodies' repair mechanisms are going to be compromised—leading to more likelihood of chronic injury and even muscle atrophy.

Since IGF-1 and GH are primarily elevated during sleep, we'll also miss out on a number of the anabolic effects of IGF-1 and GH elevation during sleep.

These hormones help us to burn body fat and build more muscle tissue, but without adequate sleep, we build less muscle and burn less fat.

Chronic sleep deprivation also can zap our focus and reduce our willpower within the weight room, making it harder to hunt out those extra reps that cause future progress.

Sleep deprivation also affects coordination and motor skills, compromising our form and making us move more clumsily.

And even worse, sleep deprivation affects our inhibition and judgment, making us less likely to form good decisions or pull back a touch once we got to .

Okay, this sounds awesome!! But how do I optimize sleep for better muscle growth.

How to Optimize Sleep for Better Muscle Growth and Fat Loss?

The sleep-optimization techniques which we are going to see is called "sleep hygiene," and therefore the idea is that the more of those things we do, the more likely we are to get an good night's sleep.

- **Go to bed early.** Rather than sleeping late at night, go to bed early enough to get good 7 – 9 hours of sleep.
- **Reduce Stress.** Reduce stress and anxiety levels, especially near your bedtime.
- **Get into the sun often.** This will assist you fall and stay asleep more easily in the dark because of increased melatonin production.
- **Don't go to bed right after eating**. It's usually best to avoid eating within two hours of getting to bed. within the final meal of the day, though, research shows that having high-glycemic

foods that are rich in carbohydrates helps people nod off more quickly because of increased melatonin production.

- **Keep your bedroom cool and dark.** It is easy to doze off into sleep if your bedroom temperature is cool and dark.

- **Have a shower at night.** Have a warm shower 30 mins before going to bed. This might help you cool your body temperature and make you quickly doze off into sleep.

- **Have a sleep routine.** Try to eat and sleep around the same time everyday, as this will help your body to adapt to your timings which makes the internal work (digestion, recovering etc..) much easier for your body.

Here is one sleep tip said by The Sleep Foundation, if you can't sleep within 20 minutes after you get into bed. Do a easy activity like reading under dim light until you start to feel drowsy.

I believe, now you know how important sleep is for muscle growth and fat burning, so get yourself a good 7 to 9 hours sleep a night.

CHAPTER 5:

Supplements For Body Recomposition

Supplementation is a supplement to food (it's even in the name) and we can achieve our goals without the use of supplementation, however there are times when it can be highly convenient. For instance; if you struggle to eat enough protein then a scoop of whey protein powder or a protein bar can be an easy way of helping you increase your protein intake.

It's important to remember that the goal should be to consume whole foods, from natural food sources wherever possible. However, there are three supplements I would recommend, and I have listed them below…

Whey Protein Powder- These can be purchased in powdered form or you can buy these in bottles from local supermarkets. Aim for 15-25 grams of protein per serving!

Protein Bars- These can be purchased online or in most supermarkets, aim for 15-20 grams of protein per serving (be careful these are high in fat/fibre).

Multivitamins- I highly recommend stocking up on some multi-vitamins, it may also be worth purchasing a vitamin D supplement, if your lacking natural sunlight. These can all be purchased via natural food stores or in supermarkets.

I see many people entering the gym for the first time in their life, with a shaker of BCAAs in their hand.

We will talk in detail about BCAAs in a chapter of this section, but keep in mind that supplementation is 5% of the whole picture. The rest 95%

is training properly, proper exercise execution, tracking your lifts, maintaining progressive overload(here is why getting a coach do your programming and guide you all along this process is important), following a proper balanced diet with the correct number of grams of protein, carbohydrates and fats.

Being in control of your daily and weekly caloric intake(you can do that with the information provided in this book, but getting someone whose job is to create diet plans for athletes, is superior to trying things out alone) so as to progress towards your goals.

Once and only once you have built this solid foundation, only then you should be thinking of what supplement I should buy next. Unless, you train, eat and sleep properly, supplements will do little for you.

Whey Protein Powder

Whey is a by-product of cheese production. It was once thrown away, but when scientists performed research on this semi-clear liquid they found that it is a great source of protein and more specifically, the amino acid leucine.

Leucine as mentioned before, is the main amino acid you should be aiming to get in your diet since it initiates muscle protein synthesis.

For this reason, whey protein is extremely popular nowadays. Whey supplements can be taken at any time of the day, to induce a spike in your amino acid levels, but it has the greatest effect when taken after your training session, since that is the point in time when your muscles are in highest need of amino acids, for tissue repair.

There is a chance that whey protein will not be easily digested by people whose body does not do well with dairy products. If that is you, you may consider another source of protein. But for the rest of the people, whey protein should be your main go-to. Whey is the way!

Casein Protein Powder

As milk coagulates it forms curds, such as the chunks in cottage cheese. These chunks contain casein. The main difference of casein and whey is that casein is a slower digesting protein, releasing amino acids into the bloodstream at a slower rate, but for a longer time.

So, which one should you use? Whey or casein? To answer that I would suggest you take whey protein(30-40grams) as your post-workout shake, since after training your muscles are in huge need of a spike in amino acids. Again supplementing with whey should be done only in cases which you are not able to eat after training. Otherwise, food can do the job for you perfectly.

Casein should be taken throughout the day, to maintain somewhat high levels of amino acid, but most importantly before bed. This is the point where casein's slow absorbance comes into play.

During sleep your body will be deprived of any amino acids for 8 or so hours. Because of casein we will be able to provide a constant slow release of amino acids for the first hours of the night.

Egg Protein Powder

In our list of protein sources, eggs (egg powder) could not be missing. Egg protein powder has a perfect PDCAA score(ranges from 0 to 1) of 1, which is the maximum! PDCAA score, Protein Digestibility Corrected Amino Acid score shows the quality of the protein, and is calculated by using humans' amino acid requirements and their ability to digest it.

Egg protein powder is derived from the egg white, which means it has neither carbohydrates nor fat. It is equally as good as whey protein in stimulating protein synthesis and has even slower absorption rate than casein.

All in all, with a PDCAA score of 1 we can not ignore egg protein powder. This protein source makes of a good supplement that can be used in cases other than the pre-workout and post-workout meals.

Soy Protein Powder

Soy protein is the most popular plant based protein powder on the shelves of supplement stores and even organic food stores. Please stay away from it. Here are a few good reasons why you should do so.

Regular intake of soy foods has feminizing effects in men due to isoflavones. Isoflavones are estrogen-like molecules found in soybeans. According to a research carried out by Harvard University, soy and isoflavones were associated with a reduced sperm count in semen.

Research done by the U.S. Department of Agriculture has also shown that soy is responsible for decreased absorption of protein and other nutrients. Also, a study has also shown that soy intake can lead to increased risk of breast cancer cell growth, for women.

Other Plant Based Proteins

Rice, pea, hemp protein powders are some plant based proteins others than soy. Rice protein has a PDCAA score of 0.47. Combining rice protein with pea protein(PDCAA score of 0.69 and high amount of leucine), makes this blend a good choice. This is actually what vegans choose when it comes to protein powder supplementation.

Hemp protein is not easily digested and should be your last choice of plant based protein. It is about 30-50% protein by weight, while other protein sources we talked about before are 90-100% protein. Even though being rich in omega-3 and omega-6 fatty acids, hemp should be avoided, since there are better choices for protein supplements in the market.

BCAA

I am sure you have seen lots of guys in your gym, carrying around a bottle or a shaker containing a pink solution. Well, these are BCAAs. BCAAs stands for Branched Chain Amino Acids. These amino acids are essential amino acids which means that your body can't produce, and for this reason you have to take them through food. These include leucine, isoleucine and valine.

Leucine is your best friend. Leucine is responsible for initiating protein synthesis and should be taken especially before and after training, as mentioned before.

Isoleucine comes second in the priority list. This amino acid improves glucose metabolism and increases its(glucose) uptake by the muscles, thus allowing for better training performance.

Valine is the 3rd and last in the list of priority of branched chain amino acids. Its effects are not nearly significant when compared to leucine and isoleucine.

There are lots of studies on the internet showing that BCAAs are responsible for improved immune function, reduced fatigue, increased muscle growth and others, and these studies are exactly the ones that supplement companies use to convince you that these supplements are worth your money.

Yes, BCAAs supplements do show all these brilliant effects, but what most studies miss is the fact that their participants are not eating properly in the first place. No attention is being paid on caloric intake and more specifically on the grams of protein consumed per day by these participants.

Of course if these athletes are under-eating protein, then taking a BCAAs supplement will have all these effects.

Your major takeaway should be that BCAAs can be equally found in food. Meat, eggs, dairy products and many other high-quality protein sources should be your BCAAs providers. All these sources contain high proportions of leucine, with a high PDCAA score.

In addition, which one do you prefer? Getting your amino acids via a shake, or eating food? Which one is more enjoyable, and also less expensive?

There is one case, though, when you should take this supplement and that is when you want to train fasted. A fasted state is a state in which your insulin levels are maintained low in your blood stream. So, you will, in other words, train with an empty stomach. The negative side to this is that it provides the perfect conditions for a negative net muscle protein balance leading to muscle loss.

The only reason one should engage in fasted training should be when training(cardiovascular training) early in the morning and have no time to eat prior to that. So, in order to prevent all that muscle breakdown I would suggest you take 10grams of BCAAS, 10-15 minutes prior to training.

In this way you can be sure that your muscle tissue will be preserved during training, while also maintaining the fasted state of low insulin levels, which according to research provides optimal conditions for fat loss.

Creatine

One of the supplements that is actually worth the investment. What most people do not know about creatine is that it is a substance naturally found in your body. Our aim with supplementing it is just to increase its amounts and thus its effects.

These include, building muscle, improved strength, reduced training-induced muscle damage and soreness and increased anaerobic endurance.

Creatine has been a subject of numerous studies. There are rumors running around, that creatine damages your kidneys. Studies have shown that short and long term usage of creatine by healthy individuals showed no kidney damage. Individuals who do suffer from kidney diseases, should not be taking creatine. Please get your medical doctor's consent before embarking on your creatine journey.

I am sure you have heard of many different kinds of creatine in the market. I know, companies always want to come up with something new so that they can price products higher. Creatine citrate, liquid creatine, creatine ethyl-ester, creatine nitrate, buffered creatine and creatine hydrochloride are just a few examples of creatine forms.

However the winner of the contest between all forms of creatine is creatine monohydrate. Regard the monohydrate form as your gold standard. Keep in mind that all other forms of creatine are compared to the monohydrate form in terms of effectiveness.

One small disadvantage of creatine monohydrate is that it is not very water soluble. In the case it effects your stomach you can consider other forms of creatine such as micronized creatine monohydrate, creatine hydrochloride or creatine citrate or nitrate. These are more water soluble.

How To Take Creatine

The most common way to load creatine is to take 20grams per day for 5-7 days, followed by a daily intake of 5grams. However, you can just take 5grams a day, every day, if you are just starting out with creatine supplementation. Keep in mind though that if you choose to go the ''loading-way'', creatine's effects will kick in faster, since more of it will accumulate in the muscles.

When Should You Take Creatine

Research shows that the most effective time to take creatine is after training, along with your post-workout meal. One research showed that taking creatine with carbohydrates, increases its absorption, since insulin levels in the blood are higher.

One study carried out by the University of Nottingham, showed that 50g of protein along with 50g of carbohydrates, had the same effect in augmentation of creatine accumulation in the muscles.

This study shows that taking creatine after training showed greater results in body composition and strength than before training. So, choose to take creatine with a nice, big, nutritious post-workout meal, rich in carbohydrates and protein.

Cycling Creatine

Do not confuse creatine with steroids. You should not cycle on and off creatine, in other words have periods when you take creatine and others when you do not. There is no scientific evidence that supports that creatine supplementation by healthy individuals is associated with any adverse effects, even with long term usage.

One more myth has been debunked here.

Creatine And Caffeine

Most pre-workout supplements contain both creatine and caffeine. They back this up by quoting a study done by the University of Luton which showed that a combination of creatine and caffeine is more effective than just creatine, on improving the performance of athletes doing HIIT training.

Another study by the University of Yu Da showed results that support the statement above.

However, there is a study by the University of Leuven that demonstrated that taking both creatine and caffeine before training, decreased muscular force production, when compared to just creatine monohydrate use.

So, as you can tell, research on this topic, shows contradicting results. I would suggest you to play it safe and just take caffeine before training and creatine after training, with your post-workout meal.

Creatine In A Cutting Phase

Creatine is highly suggested when you are cutting. It helps you retain muscle mass and preserve strength. This study backs this up. As of the bloating, due to water retention that once used to go along with creatine, do not worry about this. This is not an issue any more, since more high-tech machinery allows for better processing of creatine.

CHAPTER 6:

Maintaining your Body Muscle so you don't lose it, even over 50

Losing muscle is a scary concept, especially for those who have seen how deteriorating muscles have affected loved ones. People over the age of 50 are more prone to muscle loss. But it does not have to be your lot in life to lose muscle if you go through the proper training and keep up good habits.

Preventing Muscle Loss

The best way to maintain muscle mass is to go to the gym, but that is often easier said than done. There are so many excuses that seem logical at the time but eventually eat at your resolve to maintain a healthy level of muscle during your life. Remember, though, that you are responsible for the happiness in your own life. To prevent the deterioration of mind and body, resolve to prevent muscle mass today.

The key to maintaining muscle is to train at nearly the same levels you have in the past but take a break every once in a while. Changing your routine may seem hard at first, but it is the first step to continuing a healthy lifestyle. The majority of the hard work is already behind you, so take advantage of the gains you have made.

Weight Training for Life

If you are new to weight training, check with your doctor before starting a new routine, especially if you have an injury. Starting weight loss over the age of 50 comes with its own struggles, including loss of muscle from a sedentary life and restricted range of motion. However, that should not stop you from starting your journey. Visit a physical therapist if you continue to struggle.

Weight training is the only type of exercise that prevents the reduction of muscle mass over time. Aerobic exercise is a common go-to for many who are new to exercising because it gets your heart rate up and helps reduce weight. However, if you want to maintain muscle mass as you age, choose weight training over aerobic exercise. The best results, of course, come from incorporating a combination of the two exercises, giving you both brain and body health.

Get Enough Protein

It is important to get enough protein into your diet to account for your muscle gains. However, as you get older, ingesting enough protein is vital. The body needs the extra nutrients to build muscle and perform daily functions. It is estimated that older people need as much as 0.2 g more protein per pound than their younger counterparts.

Eat Right

The better you eat as you age, the more likely you are to maintain muscle and perform daily activities without troubles. Aim for eating foods that will give you energy. After all, these are the foods that will keep you going when you are at the gym. You are less able to metabolize nutrient-lacking food as you get older, making weight gain more common. Find the foods you like best from every category (starches, proteins, fruits, vegetables, and fats), and increase your intake.

Though it is not vital to weigh yourself every day, keeping track of your weight can help you discover how much you need to lose, and which foods work best given the amount of weight lost. If you are careful with your caloric intake, you can still lose or maintain weight while sneaking a slice of pie into your routine. If you are over 50, however, remember to decrease the total amount of fat you consume daily.

Train Right

When starting out, many people fall into the trap of working out incorrectly. Though you may see some gains from this method, it is far more likely that you will neither gain as much muscle nor lose as many calories when you perform moves incorrectly. Thankfully, modern technology has made it possible for everyone to learn how to do any workout move recorded through video. Visit YouTube to discover how to move correctly to both help you gain muscle and prevent injury.

Another solution is to hire a personal trainer. Most gyms offer a personal training program that will give you the right exercises for your body type while helping you as you work out. The advantages of personal trainers cannot be understated. They know how each movement affects the way your body moves, and they help you feel better as you work out. They will also give you tips for gaining muscle for your body type, age, and sex, all invaluable information.

Be mindful of your body and its limits while exercising. If you feel hungry or thirsty before heading to the gym, eat a small snack and drink at least two glasses of water before performing any exercises. Not only is it difficult to maintain your usual pace when your body is not fully nourished, but you may experience light headedness and cramps as well. If you feel faint while working out, stop immediately and grab a glass of water. Next time you head to the gym, be sure to eat at least four hours before exercising.

Get Enough Rest

Sleep is one of the most sought-after commodities in this fast-paced world. It is common to feel tired all the time if you are not getting enough sleep every night. So, imagine how much more detrimental the effect of little sleep has on your body if you are building muscle.

When you sleep, your body repairs the damage made to the body during weight training. The insulin-like growth factor hormone becomes active when you sleep, helping muscles repair and breaking down carbs to give you energy for tomorrow.

The quality of your sleep also determines how well you will build muscle. If you have a highly irregular sleeping pattern (going to sleep at 9 PM on Wednesday then staying out until midnight on Friday), you will not receive all the benefits that come from a regular sleeping schedule. The body loves routine, and breaking routine will often result in difficulty sleeping. Though changing the time, you go to sleep occasionally will not have a significant effect on your quality of sleep, consistently changing when you hit the sack will prevent proper muscle growth.

Limit Alcohol

Alcohol is another culprit that prevents proper sleep, ultimately leading to fewer gains (except when it comes to fat gains). Drinking a glass of wine, a couple times per week will not upset your schedule much but drinking every night will prevent you from achieving a good night's rest. Consider the last time you drank too much. Feeling hungover is a good sign that your body did not get the time it needed for repair.

Alcohol may result in muscle loss, if you are not careful. Alcohol prevents the body from producing hormones like estrogen and testosterone, which may hinder the growth of muscle.

Physique Maintenance

After you have gained muscle, it may feel like a step back to consider maintenance of that muscle, but that does not mean that you have to stop progressing. In fact, you should keep moving to see how far you can go. One of the greatest joys in life is achieving goals, and once you gain muscle, you can keep gaining muscle until you feel and look your best.

Remember, muscle maintenance does not mean giving up entirely. You may still find it useful to add weight when you train but slow down the rate of change considerably. You will also not lose muscle if you choose to take a day or two offs. Your body still works at a higher metabolic rate even after taking a week off, but do not make a habit of skipping weeks.

Nutrition

During the difficult stage of building muscle, your body constantly craves food, and intense workouts often give you the excuse to eat more. But what happens when you want to stop gaining muscle? Your caloric intake should level off, and you should be neither eating too much or too little. Use the BMR you determined in the first few chapters and stay at that steady pace.

Once you have finished pushing your body to its limits, you can start eating the foods you want again. Remember, of course, that eating the right foods and exercising consistently are the most important ways to maintain muscle, but you are no longer trying to produce massive gains. Your body does not need as much protein to maintain muscle mass. Carbohydrates are not as necessary in your diet. Find a routine that works for you and be consistent.

Supplements

Your wallet will finally thank you when you reach the muscle-maintenance level. Suddenly, you do not have to dip into your savings to buy protein powder, expensive pre-workout drinks, or muscle-building supplements like creatine. Instead, focus on keeping the supplements that give you the correct nutritional value. If you only consume a multivitamin and an iron supplement, you will stay at the same level of fitness while sustaining your diet specifications. Note: if you are a woman and no longer menstruate, often iron supplementation is not necessary. Check with your doctor.

CHAPTER 7:

Mistakes of Body Recomposition and how to avoid them

Not Consuming Enough of the Appropriate Foods.

Nutritious diets are key to that muscle mass. Don't fool yourself that you should consume anything you want. Perhaps the most rigorous workout routine is not going to make up for a bad diet. Consuming so much processed carbs and high-fat diets can prevent you from reaching your optimal physical health. And don't worry about protein — everyone is a little special, but people involved in losing weight will seek to consume their body weight in grams of protein. If you're trying to lose weight in order to hit 190 pounds that means you're going to want to achieve 190 grams of protein. If you're attempting to add weight, you're going to want to increase the number a bit.

Often Keeping to the Same Schedule

Several guys in the gym still go for the same weights, perform the same amount of sets, in the same order every time they practice. It may be harder on your head, so it's better on your body, too. If you want to see changes, perhaps you need to move away from the curves of your head. Changing the schedule would even keep you from becoming frustrated. That might mean doing something you've never done before, which may feel a little daunting. Instead of shying away from anything when you're scared, you're not going to be any luck at all, Outside Online decides it's time to pick up the task. Incorporating new movements can help avoid muscle imbalances that may contribute to injury.

Screwing up sets Even though you do the best on any move.

You won't see the outcome though you take a 10-minute break in each session. The number of sets, as well as the amount of repetitions that you do, also has a significant effect on your capacity to develop muscle. Bodybuilding.com recommends you can strive for 12 to 20 sets of 8 to 15 replicates in places where you're wanting to see progress, but you can do that for less for muscle groups where you're not aiming to develop as much. And while your ego may encourage you to hang on to the weight, it's not the best idea. You're likely to make more progress if you stay in the stable, maintain a decent form, and try for more repetitions.

4. Not having enough rest: Insufficient sleep will contribute to all kinds of health conditions, such as heart disease and diabetes. When you're not well enough, you're never going to be able to drive yourself as much as you want. For those who are dealing with insomnia, developing healthier sleeping patterns is important. Reducing the volume of caffeine, you drink in the afternoon and turning off your appliances at least one hour before you sign home. Sleep isn't the only kind of relaxation you can remember, since you can always overdo it when you get a lot of shut eye. If you visit the gym every single day for hours, that's way too many.

Overdoing Cardio

Every successful workout regimen requires a mix of aerobic workouts and power workouts. The important thing is to work out the correct mix. People trying to create muscle will totally ruin their attempts if they spend so much time on the treadmill. Men's Gym reports that going crazy on exercise workouts can deplete the accumulated calories that are required for muscle development. It's particularly dangerous if you work out on an empty stomach. The article went on to claim that this is going to cause the body to use muscle as a heat.

And how much of it is too many? It depends on the person. Natural Health means that it continues for three to four hours, running between 30 and 40 minutes. If you choose high-intensity bursts, stick to two or three hours. Even with these rules, though, you can continue to adapt to how the body responds.

CONCLUSION

Make working out a habit! Workout everyday, eat nutritious, sleep well and enjoy your transformation into whole new man/woman. Get up early in the morning and dedicate one hour to workout everyday and make that a habit — you want to train yourself to control your body and calm, tell yourself to get up but not to fall asleep! No matter what the obstacle is, you have the power to tackle it and transform yourself. You will be happy one day for taking the steps to transform yourself.

After few weeks, you might feel less motivated, stressed and lazy to getup and workout. But do not give up, you didn't start to give up right? Ignore those negative thoughts and do it anyway no matter how demotivated you are. Getting up from the bed is your first victory, you have taken control over-your body, now go and transform your life.

Concentrate on every part of your body, consciously calming your muscles. It's a field check. If you've not finished the exercises, you should continue doing them. If you feel nervous, track the level of stress during the day. When you feel stressed, take a few quick breaths, think about the term "relax," and allow your body to return to a state of relaxation.

After following all the techniques discussed in this book, I guarantee you will look and feel much better. You may have to buy new clothes. You may get compliments. You may find that you love working out. One thing you will find is that you begin to feel better and have more energy and that is the most important thing, feeling good!

Ensure that you are actually implementing the different points which you have learned in this book. We would ask you to maintain a diary which will record the whole journey. The process of losing weight is not the easiest. However, if you have done justice to the book and you actually did as we instructed, we are confident that you must look a lot slimmer and fitter than before. Fitness has a lot of perks and you need to try all you can for the sake of shedding the pounds. With this book as a guide and the right tips with you, you should face no difficulty whatsoever in attaining your goals.

At this point you should be ready and have your plan in place ready to take action. Make sure you have your motivational list of benefits stuck to the fridge in big bright letters, a new shopping list of healthy goods and an organized routine of exercise which you can add to and change around as you go along. It's helpful if you tick off any smaller goals as you progress along your weight loss journey to reach the ultimate goal of a happy and healthy life.

Remember never to give up and keep trying even if it seems hopeless. You will get the hang of it. Positivity and persistence are the key and it will unlock many things for you over time.

DO YOU WANT TO SIGN UP IN OUR 12-WEEK PROGRAM?

Do you want to get fit?
Do want to feel strong?
Do you want to wear clothes that makes you super hot? And makes you extremely sexy when you take them off?
Do you want to be a better role model for your family and friends?
Do you want to feel energetic and enthusiastic all the time?

Do you want feel confident?

But,

✘ You set a plan in January and by March you're back to square one
✘ You eat healthy most of time but then can't follow thru
✘ You can't afford a personal trainer
✘ You're not getting your monies worth from your gym membership
✘ You want to workout at your own pace
✘ You get intimidated working out with other people
✘ You get bored with your workouts

✘ You lose motivation easily

Does any of this sound like YOU?

NO PROBLEM. WE BRING THE TRAINING AND NUTRITION PLAN TO YOU!

And I am here to help you achieve your dream body and I love doing it.

LOSE THE WEIGHT AND KEEP IT OFF

UNCOVER EXACTLY HOW TO GET IN THE **BEST SHAPE OF YOUR LIFE WITH** CONSISTENT WORKOUTS. EASY TO FOLLOW NUTRITION PLAN AND

AMAZING RESULTS.

Do you want to know what you will get when you signup with us?
Do you want to know what our clients has to say?
Do you want to know what our social media connections has to say?
Check out our website [here](www.clubforfitness.com) (www.clubforfitness.com)

Signup with us and get amazing results in 12 weeks!!

BUT, WHO AM I?

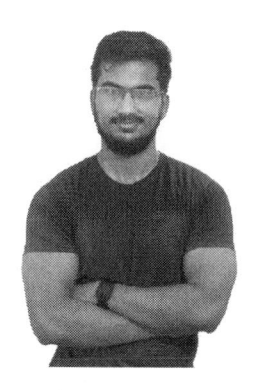

Hi, I am Charan and I am a Fitness Trainer certified by the American College of Sports Medicine.

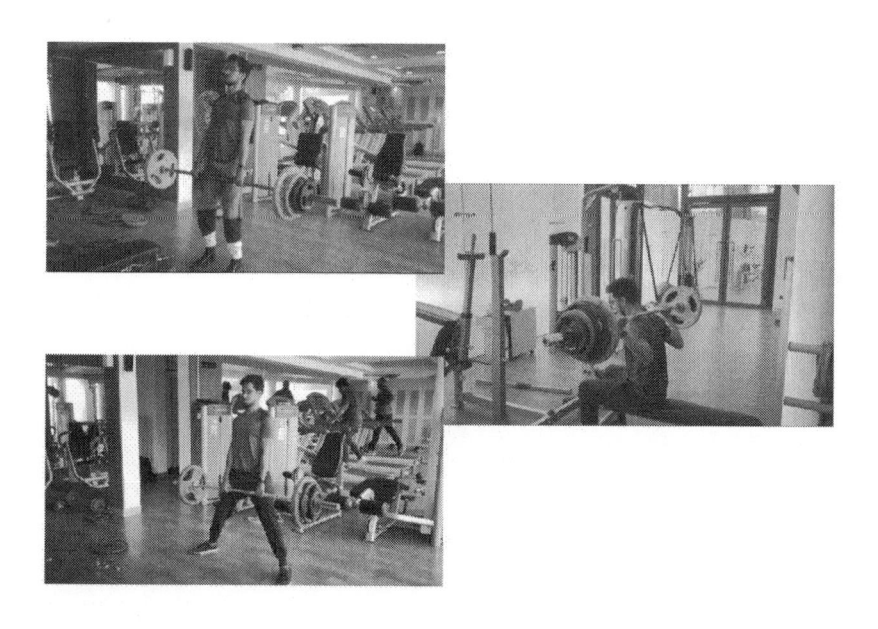

But before that, I used to be very lean and weak from my childhood till my end of my college days and then I started learning about my body, working out, eating healthy and as soon as I started developing myself in terms of physical fitness, I became stronger physically and mentally and then I figured my love and passion for fitness and I wanted to provide the same for everyone.

That's when I decided to pursue a career in fitness and start my own Online Fitness Club and later I decided to write this book on Body Recomp, because people believe that building muscle and losing fat can not be achieved at the same time and here I am to say that it is totally possible and I am going to help you achieve body recomposition with the knowledge and wisdom throughout this book.

I believe fitness is not about bulging biceps but it's about being functional. We all want to improve strength and muscle while still losing that stubborn fat, right? No worries!! Let's get started!!

Here are my social media profiles for daily valuable and amazing content:

Personal Profiles: Facebook (CharanReddyG) | Instagram (charanreddyg) | Twitter (37_charan) | LinkedIn (charan-reddy-g)

Company Profiles: Facebook (TheClubForFitness) | Instagram (clubforfitness) | Twitter (ClubForFitness) | LinkedIn (club-for-fitness)

REFERENCES

Covey, Stephen R. The 7 Habits of Highly Effective People: Powerful Lessons in Personal Change. **New York: Simon & Schuster, 2013.**

Duhigg, Charles. The Power of Habit: Why We Do What We Do in Life and Business. **New York: Random House, 2012.**

Elrod, Hal. The Miracle Morning: The Not-So-Obvious Secret Guaranteed to Transform Your Life before 8AM. **2012.**

Ferriss, Timothy. The 4-Hour Body: An Uncommon Guide to Rapid Fat-Loss, Incredible Sex, and Becoming Superhuman. **New York: Crown Archetype, 2010.**

Gawande, Atul. The Checklist Manifesto: How to Get Things Right. **New York: Picador, 2010.**

Greene, Robert. **Mastery**. New York: Penguin Books, 2013.

Holiday, Ryan. The Obstacle Is the Way: The Little Book for Flipping Adversity into Opportunity. **Penguin Group USA, 2014.**

Matthews, Michael. Bigger Leaner Stronger: The Simple Science of Building the Ultimate Male Body. **Des Moines, IA: Waterbury, 2014.**

Pilon, Brad. **Eat. Stop. Eat**. 2007.

Johnstone AM, Murison SD, Duncan JS, Rance KA, Speakman JR, Factors influencing variation in basal metabolic rate include fat-free mass, fat mass, age, and circulating thyroxine but not sex, circulating leptin, or triiodothyronine1. Am J Clin Nutr 2005; 82: 941-948.
https://www.resultswellnesslifestyle.com/blog/you-can-t-out-train-a-bad-diet

Sleep and muscle recovery: endocrinological and molecular basis for a new and promising hypothesis. https://pubmed.ncbi.nlm.nih.gov/21550729/

Juliff, L.E., Halson, S.L. (2017). Sleep, Sport and the Brain. Progressive Brain Research, 234, 13-31. doi: 10.1016/bs.pbr.2017

Mah, C. D., Mah, K. E., Kezirian, E. J., & Dement, W. C. (2011). The Effects of Sleep Extension on the Athletic Performance of Collegiate Basketball Players. Sleep, 34(7), 943-950. doi:10.5665/sleep.1132

Maxon, S. (2014, January 13). How Sleep Deprivation Decays the Mind and Body. Retrieved from https://www.theatlantic.com/health/archive/2013/12/how-sleep-deprivation-decays-the-mind-and-body/282395/

Schwartz, J., & Simon, R. D. (2015). Sleep extension improves serving accuracy: A study with college varsity tennis players. Physiology & Behavior, 151, 541-544. doi:10.1016/j.physbeh.2015.08.035

Rissa Fitness 97A Brim Boulevard Chambersburg, PA 17201

Primeval Labs: Lean Mass Recomp
https://primevallabs.com/blogs/news/body-recomposition-guide

Printed in Great Britain
by Amazon